GREAT QUESTIONS FOR NURSES TO PERSONALLY ENGAGE PATIENTS

GREAT QUESTIONS FOR NURSES TO PERSONALLY ENGAGE PATIENTS

CHAPLAIN KEITH EVANS

Contents

GREAT QUESTIONS for Nurses to Personally Engage Patients

THE GREAT QUESTIONS SERIES

GREAT QUESTIONS
For Nurses To Personally Engage Patients

The Great Questions Series
Chaplain Keith Evans

ISBN: 9798312785098
ISBN: 9798349251221

1

Introduction

A critical key to patient's feeling that their clinical healthcare was given with high-quality or not, comes through the heart of caregiver. Did the nurse, therapist or physician approach and communicate in a personal and compassionate way? Do they even care about me?

Some providers are very comfortable with initiating conversations, many others are not. They have so many intellectual responsibilities in the quality of care giving, they struggle to also give care from their hearts.

The goal of this little book is to provide a huge digest of questions that can be used as "ice breakers" that build trust and rapport but also questions to use in deepening connection and engagement with patients and families. Whether the clinician works in a private clinic, outpatient or inpatient hospital settings, there are questions that will resonate with all readers.

Are you ready to dig in and discover some wonderful questions to immediately use with patients? If so, let's go!

2

Creating Trust

Great Questions to Create Trust and Rapport

Every time we meet someone; we have an opportunity for a great first impression. If that doesn't go too well, we can have other changes – but it can be a strain. Learning some simple 'get-to-know-you' questions that are easy, open-ended and more social in nature is normally a great starting point. While this seems like common sense stuff that we each do every day – sometimes it's good to have a few more options available to break up the monotony and keep you from repeating the same question to the same person or patient a few days later.

TIPS

When appropriate and you are able, sit down when you talk or if you're doing tasks that require standing (e.g., hanging meds, assessment) - raise the bed higher so you and the patient are at closer heights. The former is scientifically proven to make the pt think you spent a lot more time with them than you did and being at similar levels provides the patient with a sense of respect/dignity.

Be situationally aware. What do you see or hear when you come into the room? Comment on the TV show they're watching or the book they're reading or the music they might be playing.

Honestly, just grab any non-medical thing they've ever mentioned and run with it. Things will flow from there.

For example, if they casually mention they have a dog, ask about their dog and other pets. If they mention they hate hospital food. Ask, "What's the first thing you want to eat when you leave?"

Key aspects of good "get to know you" questions include the following: (1,2,3, 5, 9)

- **Open-ended:** Encourage detailed answers and conversation flow. (1,2,5)
- **Variety of topics:** Cover interests, hobbies, personal values, and life experiences. (1,2,6)
- **Positive and lighthearted:** Avoid overly personal or sensitive topics initially. (1,2,5)
- **Tailored to the situation:** Adjust questions based on the setting and who you're talking to. (1,2,4)

Just listening to a patient or family member is great. Simply sharing and voicing their concerns or frustrations can be healing for them. But more social (less clinical) conversations can alleviate stress, anxiety and emotions.

There are various categories of "get to know you" questions that you can choose from, such as:

Hobbies and interests:

- Tell me something about yourself that I can't learn by reading your chart.
- How do you spend your free time?
- What's your favorite sport to watch?
- Do you play any musical instruments?
- What's your favorite type of movie genre?
- What's the last book you read that you really enjoyed?
- What's a movie you could watch every day?
- Do you have a favorite memory?
- What is your favorite TV show?
- What types of books do you like to read?
- Would you rather spend the day at a park or an art museum?
- What's one thing that can instantly make your day better?
- Do you have any pet peeves?
- Which phone app do you use the most?
- What is a skill you've always wanted to learn?

Life goals and values:

- What's your biggest accomplishment?
- What is one thing you want to achieve in the next year?
- What is your personal motto?
- What is your biggest fear?
- What do you dream about?
- What's on the top of your bucket list?

Fun and lighthearted:

- Do you have any pets?
- What's your favorite food to eat on a cheat day?
- If you could have a superpower, what would it be?
- Describe your perfect day.
- What is the worst song, in your opinion?
- What is your claim to fame?
- Do you have a morning routine?
- What's the most relaxing part of your day?
- What are you most excited about for the future?
- What do you think the ultimate theme party would be?
- What do you think the worst job out there is?
- Where is the most beautiful place you have ever seen in person?
- What's your favorite kind of weather?
- Coffee or tea?
- Do you like cities or remote places better?

- Would you survive a zombie apocalypse?
- Do you have a favorite type of exercise?
- Do you prefer cooking dinner or going out?
- Are you good at solving puzzles?
- When you are taking a shower, what do you sing?
- What's the first thing you do in the morning?

Other great "get to know you" questions: (1,2,3,4,5,7,8,9)

- What would you be doing if you weren't here at the hospital?
- What do you want to do after you get discharged?
- What's your favorite way to spend a day off?
- What was the best vacation you ever took and why?
- Where's the next place on your travel bucket list and why?
- What are your hobbies, and how did you get into them?
- Have you lived in town long?
- Do you have any brothers or sisters who live nearby? Which one is your favorite?
- What's your idea of a great weekend?
- What's your favorite place to eat around here?
- "What's your favorite way to spend a weekend?"
- "What's your dream job?"
- "Do you have any pets?"
- "What's your favorite book?"
- "What's one thing you're really passionate about?"

- "If you could travel anywhere, where would you go?"
- "What's your go-to karaoke song?"
- "What's a fun fact about you?"
- "What's your favorite thing to do in your free time?"
- "Are you a morning person or a night owl?"
- What's your favorite season and why?
- Would you rather cook or order in?
- What's your favorite board game?
- How do you prefer your coffee?
- What's your most prized possession and why?
- What would be the first thing you'd do if you won the lottery?
- How do you enjoy spending your alone time?
- What's the best concert you've ever been to?
- Ask about any upcoming holidays. Who is cooking?
- What is their favorite dish? Special recipes? Do they like leftovers?
- What was your favorite age growing up?
- What was the last thing you read?
- Which meal is your favorite: breakfast, lunch, or dinner?
- Ideally, how would you spend your birthday?
- What do you do on your commute to/from work?

3

Learning Something Personal

Great Questions to Learn Something More Personal About Your Patient

Research reveals that most patients want their providers to ask them more personal questions about their lives, beliefs and values. Often those beliefs will intersect with medical treatment options, so asking is important. But even if you do not receive a response, the patient will normally appreciate the effort.

If you are working with a patient who has difficulty opening up, try being as open-ended with your approach as possible. For example, rather than asking a pointed question, say:

- "Tell me about..."
- "I want to hear a story of..."
- "What is your opinion on..."

Great caring conversation starters: (1,2)

- What do you want me to know about you?
- Do you have any faith beliefs that might restrict medical care options (dietary, blook products, etc.)?
- How are you handling things today?
- If they've had visitors: were those friends or family?
- What do you find challenging right now? How can I support you through it?
- What do you love about life right now?
- If you could tell your younger self something you know now, what would you say?
- Have you had a significant event in your life that greatly impacted your view of the world? Would you mind sharing with me?
- Has anyone special to you died? If so, would you like to tell me about them?
- If your life slogan, what would it be?
- If your life had a soundtrack, what would it sound like?
- Tell me about times in your life when you've felt proud of yourself.
- Have you traveled much? What were some of your favorite places you've been and what did you like about them?

- What stresses you out? Do you have any pet peeves?
- If you are spiritual or religious, what does your faith mean to you? Have your beliefs changed throughout your life?
- If you could go back to school again, what would you study?
- What is the best and worst job you ever had and why?
- If you had to spend $1 million dollars tomorrow, what would you spend it on?
- What do you need today? How can I make your day a little better?
- Do you have any regrets in life?
- Do you have any fears? Have you ever had a fear that you overcame?
- What do you think has remained the same about you throughout your whole life? How have your perceptions about yourself changed over time?

Fun Personal Questions to Ask Someone (2)

- What is the biggest compliment you can give someone?
- Do you think you're a friendly person?
- What do you wish you did more of?
- What is something that makes you really angry?
- What is your biggest fear?
- How do you express your love for someone?

- What is something you consider too serious to joke about?
- What does spirituality mean to you?
- What's your least favorite emotion?
- What's your least favorite part about being you?
- How do you react to anger from others?
- What do you consider your core values?
- Do you think you have a true calling?
- Do you hold grudges, or do you let go of things easily?
- What's something that makes you envious?
- What brings you the most joy?
- What's something that makes you feel overwhelmed?
- Do you often listen to your intuition?
- Do you like small talk?
- Do you consider yourself a people pleaser?
- What's the toughest conversation you've ever had?
- What's your biggest insecurity?
- What is one thing you think most people have and never appreciate enough?
- What's the best gift you've ever received?
- Where is the fanciest place you've ever been?
- What's more important in life: excitement or stability?

4

Patient Motivations

Great Questions to Discover Patient's Motivation to Discharge

A person's values drive their decisions and motivations in life. Discovering a patient's deeper motivation can often not be what you might expect. "Getting better" is not always the answer. By learning about someone's life philosophy, you're able to get at their true essence, how they live their life, and what drives their actions.

Normally, you just can't ask, "What are your values?" That would be too abrupt, but you could curiously ask: (1)

- What do you think makes someone a "good person"?
- How do you show kindness to others?
- What do you look for in a friendship?
- What life lessons have you had to learn the hard way?

- Do you believe what is meant for you will never miss you?
- If you had only one sense (hearing, touch, sight, etc.), which would you want?
- What makes you feel at peace?
- What makes you feel most accomplished?
- Would you rather make more money doing a job you hate or less doing one you love?
- Which of your personality traits are you most proud of?
- What's the first thing you look for in a partner and/or friend?
- Do you live by any piece of advice or motto?
- How can someone earn your trust?
- How can someone lose your trust?
- Would you rather someone be honest and hurt your feelings or lie to protect them?
- If you could snap your fingers and instantly make the world better, what would you do?
- If you could only teach one thing to your (future) child, what would it be?
- Tell me a story from your childhood.

Learn more about their daily jobs and why they chose that career: (1)

- What do you/did you do for a living? What inspired you to work in that field?
- Is there one job you'd never ever do?

- What's the first thing you do after getting home from work?
- Who or what inspires you in your career?
- How do you approach taking time off from work?
- What's something an outsider wouldn't know about your industry?
- Do you have a morning routine at work? If so, what it's like?
- Are you able to work from home, and if so, do you enjoy it?
- Do you get along with all your coworkers?
- What's your favorite thing about your current job?
- What annoys you the most about your job56. What's the career highlight you're most proud of?
- What type of role do you want to take on after this one?
- Does your job make you feel happy and fulfilled? Why or why not?
- What do you remember most about your first job?
- How old were you when you started working?
- What's the worst job you've ever had?
- What originally got you interested in your current field of work?
- Are you looking forward to retiring, or do you plan to work as long as possible?
- How do you pick yourself back up after making a mistake at work?
- How do you deal with work stress?

- Who has had the biggest impact on your career choice?

Asking questions about close relationships can lead to very interesting stories, and sharing stories leads to connection and an experience of being seen and heard by one another. Try these questions:

- How much time do you spend with your family?
- Who do you most like spending time with and why?
- Which family member makes the best food?
- Which family member has had the greatest impact on you?
- What's your favorite story about your grandparents?
- What was it like growing up as the youngest/oldest/middle/only child?
- What's your favorite family memory?
- Do you ever wish you were raised differently?
- What's the best piece of advice a family member has given you?
- Do you wish you had more siblings? If so, why?
- Did you ever hide anything from or lie to your parents?
- What's your favorite way to spend time with your family?
- What's your favorite family tradition?
- What's the most important holiday you spend with your family and why?

- What's something your family would be surprised to learn about you?
- Which family member do you confide in most?
- What's more important: family or friends?
- Do you have any friends you would consider family?
- If you're married, are you close with your in-laws?
- If you're adopted, have you met any of your biological relatives?
- Would you rather go back in time to meet your ancestors, or travel to the future to meet your descendants?

5

Deeper Questions

Great Questions that Go Even Deeper

In long-term patient clinical settings or settings where you have developed a strong relationship, here are some questions that go to the next level: (1)

- What's your favorite quality about yourself? Least favorite?
- What is something that makes you feel unstoppable?
- What three words would you use to describe yourself?
- Would you call yourself brave?
- When have you felt the safest?
- What's your biggest life regret so far?
- What do you look for when finding new friends?
- Who do you admire most and why?
- Have you ever had a spiritual experience?
- What's the quickest way someone can lose your trust?

- Where is one place you've always dreamed of going?
- Is it easy for you to accept help from people?
- If money were no object, what's the first thing you would buy?
- Do you live by any particular mantra?
- If you started a business, what would it be?
- How would you spend your last day on earth?
- Do you consider yourself introspective?
- What is your number one goal in life?
- How do you hope people describe you?
- Do you want your own family someday?
- How do you see or define beauty in another person?
- Do you think dreams have deeper meanings?
- Do you often give people second chances?
- What do you think happens to us after death?
- What do you think makes someone a good person?
- What are you most grateful for in life?
- Where do you go for fresh inspiration?
- Have you ever experienced deja vu?
- What is something that gives you hope?

6

Leader Rounding Questions

Great Clinical and Leader Rounding Questions

As a provider, being personal is wonderful but remain diligent in your clinical questions. Don't just ask simple '*yes or no*' questions. (1,2,3)

Great questions for nurses to engage patients include open-ended questions that encourage conversation about their feelings, concerns, and understanding of their condition, such as:

- How are you feeling today?
- What are your biggest worries about your current situation?
- Can you tell me more about what's been happening with your symptoms?

- What are your goals for recovery?
- Do you have any questions about your treatment plan?

Key aspects of engaging patient questions:

Focus on feelings and experiences

- How does this pain feel to you?
- What are you most concerned about right now?
- Can you describe how this is impacting your daily life?

Open-ended to encourage discussion

- What questions do you have about your medication?
- Tell me about your typical routine at home.
- What are your expectations for this treatment?

Validate patient concerns

- It sounds like you're feeling frustrated with your progress.
- That's a very valid concern.
- Can you tell me more about why you're feeling this way?

Assess understanding

- Can you explain what you understand about your diagnosis?
- Do you have any questions about the instructions I've given you?
- How comfortable are you with the plan we've discussed?

For new patients

- What brought you to the hospital today?
- What is your medical history like?
- What are your hopes for this visit?

For chronic conditions

- How have you been managing your condition lately?
- Are there any changes you've noticed in your symptoms?
- What strategies have worked well for you in the past?

For discharge planning

- What are your biggest concerns about going home?
- Do you have any questions about your medications?
- Who can support you at home with your care?

Important considerations: (1,2,3)

- **Active listening:** Pay close attention to verbal and non-verbal cues to fully understand the patient's perspective.
- **Empathy:** Show genuine concern and understanding for the patient's situation.
- **Respectful language:** Use clear, simple terms and avoid medical jargon when necessary.

Great Leader-to-Nurse Rounding Questions: (5)

- In what ways can I support you in managing the stress that comes with our work here in the ______ Department?
- Are you aware of anything that may pose a safety risk to our patients, employees, or visitors?
- In what ways can I be more effective in how I provide employees with feedback?
- How can I demonstrate helping to balance your job and your personal life?
- I always want to be improving my leadership; can you tell me one thing I could do differently?
- Tell me about a co-worker who has done something you would define as excellent?
- What are the top 1 or 2 things that makes it difficult to perform your job?
- How can I demonstrate conflicts are resolved fairly in our department?

- I want to make this an organization you never want to leave, what would make this the best work environment?
- How am I doing communicating things to you?
- Give me one reason you like to work here?
- What motivates you to do your best work?
- What are suggestions for me when I need to deliver difficult information that directly impacts some or all of you?
- I want you to feel acknowledged for your hard work and contributions to the team; in what ways can I be more effective in providing feedback?
- With performance appraisals coming up, I want this performance review to feel like it will help you improve. Does the feedback I already provide enhance your performance? What can I add to improve this process?
- What skills would you like to develop further and how can I best support you in learning those skills?
- What are some ways in which employees should handle a conflict that arises between them? In what specific ways can I be more effective in addressing work-related or personality conflicts in the department?
- What can we add to the performance review process to improve the process?
- Tell me how this organization, I, and/or your peers can encourage you to be "all in" and engaged in enriching every life we serve?

- Tell me how this organization can inspire you to do your best?
- What steps can we take to achieve balance between our work and personal lives?
- How can this organization demonstrate abusive behavior is not tolerated? And Do you feel like abusive behavior has been directed towards you?
- What's not going well; what keeps you up at night concerning our patient care or safety?
- How can I (or the department) help you to better perform/succeed in your job so we always provide outstanding patient care?
- What suggestions do you have to improve cooperation/coordination, working relationships with staff from other hospital units?
- How can I (this organization or department) help you deal with stress and burnout?
- If you were running our department, what would you do differently?
- Are you getting the appropriate resources from me? Is there anything I can do differently to support you?
- What can I do to clearly demonstrate that I have your well-being and best interests in mind?
- Do you feel you know what is required to perform well in your job?
- Can you describe a recent situation in which our department members worked well together...to serve a patient? To fix a problem? Or improve something?

- What ideas do you have to improve and enhance patient outcomes, safety, and satisfaction?
- Who can I reward for demonstrating our behavioral standards?
- What professional growth or educational opportunities would you like to see for the organization or department?
- As our work lives only get busier, self-care will become an ever more important part of being authentic and having a positive impact without sacrificing our health or relationships. How are you incorporating self-care in your day-to-day work life?
- Is there anything we can do better? (process or system problems that need to be fixed?) Ideas to fix?
- Is there anything getting in the way of giving the kind of care you want to your patients?
- As your leader what do I need to start doing? And what do I need to stop doing?
- Do you feel you know the value you bring to the workplace? If so, why or why not? Please share your qualities and attributes that contribute to our success.
- Tell me about a time when you felt the suggestions were heard in the department. How can I continue to repeat the experience you just described?
- What have I done to help you do your job better? What have I done to hinder your job performance?
- What accomplishments are you most proud of? In which areas would you like to improve?

7

Conclusion

I hope you see the benefit of using these great questions with your patients. Using them will allow you as a nurse to better engage and connect to patients at a deeper, personal level.

I challenge you for the next four weeks to write down 2-3 questions to use each week with your patients and then reflect on their responses. Over a month, I'm sure you will have some amazing conversations, which certainly will increase the quality of your patient's experience while under your compassionate care.

Blessings for all that you do in your noble and sacred calling of nursing.

- - Chaplain Keith Evans

8

References

Chapter 2

1. https://www.calm.com/blog/questions-to-ask-to-get-to-know-someone
2. https://www.betterup.com/blog/questions-to-ask-to-get-to-know-someone
3. https://www.signupgenius.com/groups/getting-to-know-you-questions.cfm
4. https://www.joinonelove.org/learn/10-perfect-questions-to-ask-on-the-first-date-to-really-get-to-know-someone/
5. https://medium.com/the-ascent/50-questions-to-ask-someone-instead-of-how-are-you-9cddc96ccb86
6. https://www.panoramaed.com/blog/get-to-know-you-questions-for-students
7. https://www.womenshealthmag.com/life/ a22500573/questions-to-ask-to-get-to-know-someone

8. https://accelerate.uofuhealth.utah.edu/ improvement/nurse-leader-rounding-how-to-ask-open-ended-questions
9. https://www.teenvogue.com/story/questions-to-get-to-know-someone

Chapter 3

1. https://www.storiicare.com/blog/caring-conversation-starters
2. https://www.teenvogue.com/story/questions-to-get-to-know-someone

Chapter 4

1. https://www.teenvogue.com/story/questions-to-get-to-know-someone

Chapter 5

1. https://www.teenvogue.com/story/questions-to-get-to-know-someone

Chapter 6

1. https://accelerate.uofuhealth.utah.edu/improvement/nurse-leader-rounding-how-to-ask-open-ended-questions

2. https://www.ncbi.nlm.nih.gov/books/NBK590036/table/ch2communication.T.therapeutic_communica/
3. https://guides.libraries.psu.edu/c.php?g=319063&p=5197309
4. https://www.sanctuarypersonnel.com/blog/2020/07/five-common-nursing-interview-questions
5. https://www.capstoneleadership.net/wp-content/uploads/2022/01/Leader-Rounding-Questions-ExamplesBOSCOBEL.docx.pdf

9

THE GREAT QUESTION SERIES

Great Questions To Ask Employees
Great Questions For Spiritual Conversations
Great Questions For Nurses To Personally Engage Patients
Great Questions To Ask People With Dementia

www.ingramcontent.com/pod-product-compliance
Lightning Source LLC
LaVergne TN
LVHW022032200926
848481LV00007B/2653